The Low Carbohydrate Diet For Triathletes

by Ben Greenfield

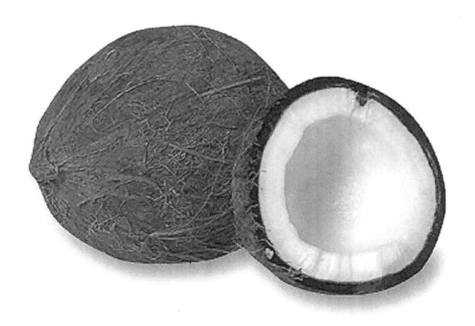

Official Nutritional Guide to Optimum Performance
For Endurance Athlete

Introduction

I bet I know what you're thinking.

If you burn a significant number of carbohydrates during endurance exercise (and you do), then how on earth can it be beneficial to consume a low carbohydrate diet?

In the first few pages of this guide, you'll not only learn why a low carbohydrate diet may be the smartest nutritional change you'll ever make in your training program, but you'll also find out why a high carbohydrate diet may be hampering your performance, your health and your longevity.

Next, you'll find out how to answer to common objections your friends and training partners will probably throw your way once you begin a low carbohydrate diet, such as "isn't carbohydrate and glucose necessary for energy?", "if you replace carbohydrate by eating more fat, won't your cholesterol increase?" and of course, the ever popular "how the heck are you going to carbohydrate load?".

Then you'll get an overview of the low carbohydrate diet for triathletes. Specifically, you'll learn proper carbohydrate, fat and protein percentages (prepare to be shocked), how to incorporate carbohydrate cycling so you don't bonk during long training sessions, and the basic foods and dietary supplements you'll need to have sitting around your kitchen.

Finally, after reviewing your grocery shopping list, we'll launch into the meat of the diet (pun intended), in which you'll find out how to eat a low carbohydrate diet for a regular week of training, for a race week and for race day.

So what qualifies *me* to tell *you* how to eat a low carbohydrate diet?

First, and probably not too importantly, I am a sports nutritionist and exercise physiologist with many years of experience coaching triathletes and tweaking the diets of elite athletes to weekend warriors.

Second, and more importantly, I have successfully incorporated this diet into my own training, as well as the programs of the athletes I coach, and found incredible success in well-being, energy, gastrointestinal function, training sessions and race day performance. In other words, I'm not just spewing out a regurgitated form of the Atkins diet – but instead giving you a nutrition plan that has been formed through testing, experimentation and a lot of significant tweaks.

So are you ready to defy the paradigm of how 99% of the sporting world is eating and learn a nutritional approach that is going to revolutionize your training and your health? Let's jump in.

Ben Greenfield

Why Choose Low Carbohydrate?

I do not recommend a low carbohydrate diet for everyone, and I especially do not recommend it for athletes who are in training phases for which they are undergoing long hours of higher intensity training (such as a professional Ironman triathlete). But there are three categories of endurance athletes who would benefit from choosing a low carbohydrate diet:

1) *Athletes trying to lose weight.*

A key component of weight loss is tapping into storage fat (adipose tissue) for energy. This fat access simply cannot happen if the body is constantly drawing on carbohydrate reserves and blood glucose for energy. In a moderate to high carbohydrate diet, not only does the utilization of fat for energy become far less crucial, but the body never becomes ideally efficient at using fat.

There is a growing body of evidence that a high fat, low carbohydrate diet causes faster and more permanent weight loss than a low fat diet. Furthermore, appetite satiety and dietary satisfaction are significantly improved with a high fat, low carbohydrate diet that includes moderate protein intake.

My own personal experience with a low carbohydrate diet began with an off-season attempt to lose holiday fat pounds, followed by the stark realization that contrary to my expectations and what I had been taught in traditional sports nutrition classes, my performance and energy levels actually improved despite a lower carbohydrate intake.

2) *Athletes wanting to improve health and longevity.*

When glucose is used to create energy, a high number of free radicals are produced. Free radicals are dangerous molecules that can damage normal cellular processes. The burning of fat for energy does not create this same cellular damage. In an endurance athlete who is already creating a high number of damaging free radicals from exercise, further damage from high blood glucose levels becomes a nasty one-two combo.

In addition, the constantly elevated levels of circulating blood sugars that can be caused by a moderate to high carbohydrate diet are associated with nerve damage, small dense cholesterol particles (the culprits for heart disease), high morbidity, bacterial infection, cancer progression and Alzheimer's.

As you will learn later in this guide, simply getting these your energy levels from non-blood glucose based energy sources can directly improve your quality of life, and allow you to ensure that you live longer and healthier.

3) *Athletes who have consistently poor performance or gastrointestinal distress while training or racing.*

Because of genetic predispositions, some athletes are much more sensitive to the fluctuations in blood sugar caused by carbohydrate intake. Often, the result of this sensitivity is a short-lived initial increase in energy levels after consumption of a sports bar, sports drink, gel or other carbohydrate source, following by a sharp and drastic drop in energy levels. But the calories from fats and proteins are utilized at far more stable rate than carbohydrate sugar, resulting in more stabilized energy levels.

In addition, uncomfortable amounts of gas and bloating in the endurance athletes can be due to the high rate of bacterial activity caused by carbohydrate fermentation in the digestive tract. Many athletes experience an even greater degree of gastrointestinal distress from food allergies or intolerances to common carbohydrate sources, particularly wheat.

So who should *not* choose a low carbohydrate diet?

First, endurance athletes in the heat of competition, such as during an Ironman triathlon, will certainly need a higher carbohydrate intake than appears in the typical training week meal plan in this guide. But that's why there is also a race day plan included!

Next, endurance athletes going through an extremely heavy block of training *that is a higher load to which they are accustomed*, such as a triathlon camp that involves 25-40 hours of training per week, will also need a higher carbohydrate intake (although this volume of training and carbohydrate intake is not healthy, it is a necessary sacrifice for injecting large doses of endurance into the body).

Finally, individuals with diseases or conditions that disable the ability to properly metabolize fats and proteins (such as gallbladder removal) may also need to eat a higher percentage of daily calories from carbohydrates.

Answering Objections

Once your training partners, family or other friends learn that you're eating fewer carbohydrates, you're guaranteed to hear several objections and see some raised eyebrows. Typically, the criticism of a low carbohydrate diet falls into three categories of questions:

Objection #1: Isn't glucose and carbohydrate necessary for energy during exercise?

As mentioned earlier in this guide, directly burning blood glucose for fuel causes a significant amount of free radical damage compared to burning storage carbohydrate, storage fats, or circulating fats in the bloodstream. This type of fuel utilization occurs in the endurance athlete trained to eat a gel every 20 minutes during every single training session, or to constantly have sports drink on the edge of the pool and a bowl of pasta waiting at home to re-fuel after the workout.

While cells can certainly burn glucose for energy, fat is a preferred energy source in nearly every cell, and especially for the mitochondria, which are the energy-creating organelles within most cells. Until extremely high exercise intensities are achieved (rarely the case among endurance athletes) or until the human body has exercised for 2-3 hours continuously, fat is completely useable as an energy source. Specifically, natural saturated fats, omega-3 fatty acids, and medium chain triglycerides are extremely dense energy sources that produce very little damaging byproducts from their metabolic use for energy.

The specific parts of the body that do need glucose on daily basis are the brain, the nerves, special proteins called "glycoproteins" (which form compounds such as mucus), and cells within the immune system, the gastrointestinal tract and the kidneys. But the total daily amount of glucose calories required by these parts of the body is about 500-700 carbohydrate calories, and not the 1500-2000 carbohydrate calories consumed by most endurance athletes!

Objection #2: Isn't fat dangerous for cholesterol-related heart disease, as well as increased risk of weight gain?

No. Not only does a high fat, low carbohydrate diet perform better for weight loss compared to a low fat, high carbohydrate diet, but there is no evidence that the cholesterol particles derived from fat increase risk of heart disease – unless fat consumption is paired with a moderate to high intake of starchy, sugary carbohydrate sources. It is at that point that cholesterol can become oxidized and lead to risk of heart disease.

The entire idea that high cholesterol causes heart disease is a flawed hypothesis, and entire books have been written on it. A very good place to start your journey into learning about the positive and healthy properties of fats would be the website http://www.cholesterol-and-health.com/ (which is in no manner affiliated with this guide – it is simply a helpful resource).

Objection #3: Don't you need to load with carbohydrate before a race?

Once you begin eating a low carbohydrate diet, your body will, within 2 weeks, become extremely efficient at burning fat. This means that you will need relatively fewer carbohydrates during race week or the day before a race, since your body develops an enhanced ability to conserve storage carbohydrate (glycogen) and also an increased ability to utilize fat as a fuel, both during rest and on race day.

What this means is that an entire week of carbohydrate loading and high sugar intake will not be necessary, and if your goal is weight loss, health, or longevity, may actually end up doing more harm than good. Since I have shifted to a lower carbohydrate intake, I have found that the 85-90% carbohydrate diet I was eating during race week is no longer necessary. The primary changes made during race week are A) a carbohydrate dense breakfast the day before and the morning of the race; and B) frequent snacking in the last several days leading up to the race (not allowing a feeling of hunger to set in). This would still be considered "carbohydrate loading", but not in the common tradition of loading, which typically includes 7-10 days of high carbohydrate intake before an event.

Low Carbohydrate Diet Overview

The average endurance athlete eats a diet of about 50-60%+ carbohydrate, 20-30% protein and 20-30% fat. As I talk about in my book "Holistic Fueling for Ironman Triathletes", the problem with this type of dietary intake is not necessarily the percentages (unless you are indeed trying to eat a low carbohydrate diet), but instead the source from which many of these foods are commonly derived – from sources such as cookies, crackers, pasta, biscotti, scones, bagels, muffins, energy bars, juice, processed trail mixes, etc. Each of these foods and others like them are very high in vegetable oils, inflammatory omega-6 fatty acids, preservatives, processed ingredients, potential food allergens, and refined sugars.

The low carbohydrate diet for triathletes addresses these issues, and includes the following components:

Higher Fat Percentage: With a macronutrient percentage of closer to *50-60% fat, 20-30% carbohydrate and 20-30% protein*, the low carbohydrate diet not only naturally eliminates many of the unhealthy food ingredients present in a higher carbohydrate diet, but also introduces more stable energy levels, less inflammation, and better weight loss. While the lower carbohydrate percentages will not sustain heavy bouts of high intensity exercise, they are perfect for lasting health, longevity, weight loss, or elimination of digestive issues from food intolerances.

Note that the percentages listed above are not a "ketogenic" diet (pure fatty acid utilization). Ketogenesis can be difficult and uncomfortable for most, and is not extremely practical from a social eating perspective either. But for a ketogenic diet, you'd be closer to 80-85% fat, 10-15% protein and 5-10% carbohydrate.

Carbohydrate Cycling: If long term carbohydrate deprivation and depletion of storage carbohydrate levels are accompanied by frequent bouts of trainings, then the immune system can eventually become depressed, physical performance and mood can decline, and risk of overtraining can increase. For this reason, storage carbohydrate should be "re-loaded" once per week, preferably on a higher volume training day during which the increased carbohydrate intake will be less damaging to the body. The meal plan in this guide is a 6 day low carbohydrate, 1 day moderate-to-high carbohydrate diet, and the higher carbohydrate intake day should preferably be the hardest day of the week (which is typically a Saturday or Sunday for most endurance athletes).

Fasted Sessions: If the goal is weight loss, then more rapid fat burning results can be attained by including fasted morning exercise sessions in this program. To implement these, simply wake up in the morning without eating anything (coffee is fine) and then engage in 30-60 minutes of exercise. It is preferable that the exercise be an easy aerobic session, since hard training sessions are more difficult to do on an empty stomach, and may result in "junk" training. Usually, an easy swim, easy bike ride, yoga session, or even a walk with the dog is sufficient. If working out in a fasted state is not possible, then it would be preferable to include longer fasted session, in which dinner is completed 3-4 hours prior to bedtime, and then breakfast is eaten 1-2 hours after waking, which, with 7-8 hours of sleep, can result in an 11-14 hour fast. You do not need to include fasted workout sessions or fasts every day of the week. I personally include these sessions 2-3 times per week, and my clients who are attempting more rapid fat loss will included these sessions 5-6 times per week.

Carbohydrate Intake During Long Workouts:

This is where things get interesting, because there are two options.

Option 1: Some people like to "train low-race high" with respect to carbohydrates. This is what I've personally done for the past several years. It means I train low carbohydrate most of the time, but actually use a large number of carbohydrates during the actual race.

If you use this approach, your gut needs to be trained to absorb as many calories as it will be taking in on race day, so if you are a Half-Ironman or

Ironman athlete, at least once every two weeks, one of your long workouts (typically the bike or run) will need to be accompanied by the use of gels, sports drinks, bars or other carbohydrate sources. Although volume will highly vary depending on size and training status, calorie intake for these carbohydrate fueled long workouts for males will be 300-450 calories per hour on the bike and 200-300 calories per hour on the run, and for females will be 250-400 calories per hour on the bike and 150-250 calories per hour on the run. All your other long workouts can be minimally fueled, with 1/2 to 1/4 as many calories as you plan on consuming on race day, and you do not need to fuel at all during any workouts that are an hour or less.

Option 2: Train low-race low. This approach involves minimum carbohydrate utilization during training (similar to option 1), but also includes minimal carbohydrate utilization during the actual event as well. The advantage is that this is a good solution if you're eating low carb for health reasons, or you if you have lots of difficult with "energy highs and lows" from typical sports gels and drinks, or you simply have lots of stomach distress from all those fermentable simple carbohydrates in typical sports gels and drinks.

The disadvantage is that it can be hard to push yourself really hard if you're not taking in many carbohydrates during a high intensity event, and for someone who is, for example, attempting to do a Half Ironman in 5 hours or less or an Ironman in 10 hours or less, the intensity is high enough to where "racing low carbohydrate" may not be realistic. You would actually have to experiment during the race to see if it works for you, and at the time of this writing, there are no athletes going at that intensity for that period of time on low carbohydrate (I'm personally experimenting with that approach during the next race season, however, and will update this book with those results and feedback).

However, if you're staying purely aerobic during your race, and not "redlining", this approach can work. It's simple, really. Here's what you do:

30-60 minutes prior to the race: 1g sodium (i.e. a chicken boullion cube – this keeps your blood pressure high enough on a low carb intake), 5-10g BCAA's or EAA's (I recommend 10 Master Amino Pattern capsules - MAP) and 2-3 tablespoons medium chain triglyceride oil or coconut oil.

Every hour during event: 5g BCAA's or EAA's (such as 5 MAP capsules per hour) and 100-150 calories UCAN SuperStarch per hour. Also - optional, but discussed more in the supplementary chapter at the end of this book - 1 serving VESPA per hour.

Basic Food Overview: Since you'll be eating a high percentage of fats, your kitchen will be stocked with coconut milk, coconut oil, coconut shavings, avocadoes, olives, extra virgin olive oil, macadamia nuts, pumpkin seeds, walnuts, sardines, salmon cheese, heavy cream, whole fat yogurt and fatty cuts of beef. For added protein, you'll also have eggs and chicken. Carbohydrate sources will be clean-burning, easily-digested fuels, including sweet potato, yam, white rice, brown rice, and fruit. Liberal consumption of non-starchy vegetables is also included.

Supplements: Your supplementation protocol should include four basic foundation supplements that are highly beneficial for health and performance: Vitamin D, magnesium, fish oil and a greens powder or greens capsule. A multi-vitamin will not be necessary if these supplements are consumed simultaneous to the rest of the foods on the plan. For added digestive health, you should include probiotics and digestive enzymes (both optional). For added performance, you can include a full-spectrum antioxidant, and for added recovery, you can include a glucosamine-chondroitin, whole amino acid, and proteolytic enzyme supplement (all optional). There is more on supplementation in the supplementary chapter at the end of this book.

The next several pages will introduce you to the grocery shopping, then your meal plan for a regular week of training, a fueling plan for long workouts, a race week meal plan and a race day meal plan.

Please be warned that as you make the transition to a low-carbohydrate diet, you will go through a period of "ketoadaptation", during which your body becomes accustomed to burning fatty acids as a primary fuel. Depending on how high your carbohydrate intake was prior to embarking upon this low carbohydrate dietary approach, you will go through a period of low energy, fatigue, grumpiness and subpar workout performance for anywhere from 4 days to 2 weeks.

This drop in energy is completely normal, and will subside after at least 2 weeks. Consider yourself warned, and as you have probably guessed, you should not switch to this diet if you are 2 weeks or less away from an important race or competition.

Many people find that adding an extra 2-3 grams of sodium per day can help tremendously with this low energy, since part of it is due to a drop in blood pressure as your body sheds carbohydrates and water.

What About When You Do Need To Eat Carbohydrates From Grains & Legumes?

As a triathlete or active endurance athlete, it can be really difficult sometimes to actually get all the carbohydrate that you need from just fruit and potatoes. Not only can that lead to "food boredom", but it can sometimes be tough or inconvenient to find these foods when you're traveling to races or at restaurants.

So although "safer starches" like sweet potatoes, yams or fruit are better choices when you need to load up on carbohydrates for a workout or race, here is what you should do if you do need to choose alternative forms of carbohydrate like grains or legumes.

1) Avoid Wheat, Soybeans and Peanuts. You can listen to my interview with Dr. William Davis to learn more about why to avoid wheat, but of all the grains, wheat is the most likely to cause rapid spikes in blood sugar and some serious digestive and gastrointestinal damage that can lead to immune system and performance problems. Most whole grain, whole wheat, and "healthy" packaged starches use wheat as a primary ingredient, so be careful! In addition, compounds called phytic acids

can bind to minerals and inhibit absorption of the compounds necessary for optimum performance. Soybeans are very high in phytates as are peanuts (although phytates in soy can be significantly reduced through fermentation, which is why fermented soy such as miso, natto and tempeh is OK, while unfermented sources such as tofu, soymilk, or edemame is not).

2) Soak & Sprout. Legumes, grains, nuts, and seeds have developed a natural protection against consumption by animals. This protection, which includes elements like "saponins and "phytic acids" allows them to resist digestion or irritate an animal's digestive system so that the legume, grain, nut or seed can bypass digestion and be "deposited" to grow elsewhere. This is an unpleasant paradox, but humans are smarter than plants and by soaking and sprouting we can cause germination, which disables these protective mechanisms in the legume, grain, nut or seed. Even if you don't sprout these foods, which is the ideal way to go, you can still soak them. Here is a great, free tutorial on soaking beans, legumes, grains, nuts and seeds.

Here is another great, free tutorial that will show you exactly how to sprout – which will allow you to eat foods like quinoa, amaranth, millet, or even "safer" forms of wheat like Einkorn wheat berries without the digestive issues or risk.

By avoiding wheat, soybeans and peanuts, and actively soaking and sprouting your beans, legumes, grains, nuts and seeds, you open yourself up to being able to consume a larger variety of carbohydrates for those times when you actually do need more carbohydrates, such as during a race week, or on the day of a very hard or long workout.

Grocery shopping list

Carbohydrate sources are:

- Sweet Potato and/or Yam (these are considered starchy vegetables)
- White Rice, Brown Rice and/or Quinoa
- Gluten free bread or wrap
- Organic Fruit (you can choose your favorites, but good ones are raspberries, papaya, banana, strawberries, peaches)
- Organic Vegetables:
    - Cabbage
    - Butter lettuce leaves
    - spinach
    - kale, bok choy, and/orswiss chard
    - broccoli
    - cauliflower
    - Brussels sprout
    - bell peppers
    - nori (seaweed)
    - Sauerkraut
    - Garlic
    - Cucumber
    - Crimini mushrooms
    - Red onions
    - Green onions
    - Parsley
    - Zucchini
    - Shallots
    - Sugar snap peas
    - Cilantro

- Bean sprouts

Protein sources are:

- Wild Atlantic salmon
- Herring
- Anchovies
- Cod
- Shrimp
- Organic grass fed beef (choose fattier cuts)
- Organic free range chicken
- Omega 3 enriched eggs from free range chickens

Fat sources (in addition to proteins listed above) are:

- Macadamia nuts
- Brazil nuts
- Almonds
- Pumpkin seeds
- Walnuts
- Hemp seeds
- Sesame seeds
- Avocadoes
- Olives
- Coconut Oil
- Whole Coconut milk
- Unsweetened Coconut shavings
- Whole Greek yogurt
- Feta cheese
- Cocochia bars/snack mix

Beverages:

- Kombucha
- Teeccino

Condiments:

- Ghee (clarified butter) if you can get at grocery store
- Lemon juice
- Extra virgin olive oil
- Apple cider vinegar
- Rice vinegar
- Sesame oil
- Non-soy soy sauce alternative
- Minced garlic
- Capers
- Lemon
- Water Chestnuts
- Ginger
- Cayenne Pepper
- Fish sauce
- Wasabi

Additional recommendations:

LivingFuel SuperGreens Meal Replacement. If you must get quick nutrition and don't have time to cook, 2-3 heaping scoops of the Living Fuel SuperGreens mixed in ½ cup whole coconut milk or water can be used as a meal replacement for ANY of the meals on this plan. For an even lower carbohydrate option, such as when you are sitting at the office or late at night, the same substitution can be made, but with <u>Living Fuel SuperProtein</u>.

Meal Plan For Regular Training Days

This is the meal plan that you will stick to for 6 days of each week (remember that there is still 1 day per week that will involve a higher carbohydrate intake). For each meal, choose one option. If you are a male or a large person, choose the higher range of caloric volume (i.e. if it says 2-3 eggs, eat 3, or it says one medium-large sweet potato, choose large).

Breakfast (choose 1) – Whenever possible, complete any of your easy workouts in the morning, before breakfast. For added benefit, do not eat within 2 hours of bedtime.	-Eggs: 2-3 eggs with one medium-large sweet potato or yam. Scramble eggs in coconut oil or ghee with mix of your choice of vegetables, and serve with sea salt, black pepper, and 1 fried or baked sweet potato, yam or taro. Serve with liberal amount of steamed vegetables of choice, and top with feta cheese. -3/4-1 cup whole coconut milk blended with ice, cinnamon and 1 handful blueberries or chopped/sliced fruit of choice. -2-3 scoops Living Fuel Supergreens with 1 packet Cocochia mix or 1 handful macadamia nuts or Brazil nuts -3/4-1 cup whole Greek yogurt with 1

	handful macadamia nuts and 1-2 handfuls or chopped/sliced fruit of choice Limit coffee/caffeine intake to no more than equivalent of 8-12 ounces black coffee or tea. It would be fine (and actually encouraged) to drink one to two cups of <u>Teeccino</u> per day.
Snack 1	No mid-morning snack necessary on any day *except* the hardest workout day of the week – in which case you'll be using the next meal plan (don't worry, infrequent eating doesn't cause your metabolism to drop). If you get extremely hungry between breakfast and lunch, have a couple tablespoons of coconut oil.
Lunch	Large vegetable salad. You can chop and serve as many non-starchy vegetables as you'd like, salt and pepper to taste, and drench in 3-4 tablespoons extra virgin olive oil or macadamia nut oil, and apple cider vinegar. Include 2 handfuls black olives, 1-2 handfuls pumpkin seeds and ½-1 sliced avocado. Alternatively, you can have leftovers from the previous night's dinner – which you'll end up doing quite often.
Dinner	

-2-3 eggs and ½-1 avocado, chopped and sautéed in coconut oil and wrapped in kale, bok choy, swiss chard, or cabbage leaf. Salt and pepper to taste. (do not eat this if you had eggs for breakfast already). Alternatively, instead of using eggs + avocado, you can use 6-9 oz of herring or anchovies to fill wrap. Serve with a ¾-1 cup of cooked White Rice, Brown Rice and/or Quinoa, mashed sweet potato, yam or taro. For a starch substitute you can also do <u>sweet potato fries</u>

-6-9oz salted beef or salmon. Rub with minced garlic and serve with lemon juice and as many non-starchy vegetables as you'd like, steamed or sautéed, and lightly salted. Season with salt, pepper, kelp, kombu, and/or dulse seasoning. Serve with a ¾-1 cup of cooked White Rice, Brown Rice and/or Quinoa, mashed sweet potato, yam or taro.

-6-9oz chicken. Prepare as desired and serve with 1/2-1 avocado, and as many non-starchy vegetables as you'd like, steamed or sautéed, and lightly salted. Season with salt, pepper, kelp, kombu, and/or dulse seasoning. Serve with a ¾-1 cup of cooked White Rice, Brown Rice and/or Quinoa, mashed sweet potato, yam or taro.

-<u>Spicy Shrimp & Onions.</u> ←click for video. Use 6-9 large shrimp and serve with a ¾-1ncup of cooked White Rice, Brown Rice and/or Quinoa, mashed sweet potato, yam or taro.

-Chicken skewers with almond sauce. This is a more family style recipe, so volume will depend on the number of people you're feeding, but you should eat the equivalent of two small-medium breasts, with 1-2 tablespoons of the almond sauce. Cut chicken breasts in 1/2 thickness strips. Marinate in non-soy soy sauce alternative for about 2 hours. BBQ chicken on skewer or bake at 350 until cooked through. Plate on a big bed of spinach.

Almond Sauce

> 1/4 creamy Almond Butter
> 2 tsp honey
> 2 tsp non-soy soy sauce alternative
> 1 Tbl brown rice vinegar
> 2 tsp grated ginger
> 1/2 cup coconut milk

Combine all ingredients in a sauce pan over medium heat. Cook until thickens - about 5 min.

-Cod Dish

1 tsp olive oil or macadamia oil (more heat stable)
2 Cod fillet (you can multiply this recipe by the number of people you're feeding, but you eat the equivalent of 1 medium-large fillet)
2 Tbl unsalted butter or ghee or coconut oil
3 Tbl salted capers
a handful of fresh parsley, finely chopped
one lemon

Drizzle olive oil or macadamia oil on to the fish fillets and season with salt and pepper. Gently heat a non-stick frying-pan and add the fish, skin down, and cook until the skin starts to color and turn golden and crisp. Turn up the heat slightly and add the fresh butter and after a couple of minutes, turn the fish over. Finish cooking until the butter begins to turn brown (be careful not to let it go black). Add the capers, chopped parsley and finish with a good squeeze of lemon juice to deglaze the pan. Remove the fish from the pan and serve immediately.

Serve with roasted veggies/potatoes

3 sweet potatoes halved
1 Bell pepper cut in 1/2 in cubes
1 onion quartered
1 zucchini cubed
1/4 Cup balsamic vinegar
2 Tbl olive oil
1 tsp salt
Black pepper

Before roasting, boil potatoes for 20 min. or until potatoes can easily be pierced with a fork. Eat the equivalent of ¾-1 cup of this.

-Miracle Noodles with Chicken <u>(this is just one example of a good Miracle Noodles recipe – more on their website – big fan of these, to read why click here):</u> Cook 150-250 calories miracle noodles according to package directions. Meanwhile, sautee sliced chicken breast in 1 tsp. olive oil, with red bell 1/2 of a chopped cucumber, a handful of sliced red onions, a handful of sliced mushrooms, a handful of chopped broccoli, and handful of spinach, and 1 crushed garlic clove. Serve over miracle noodles. This meal is slightly lower calorie, and would be best for a completely easy or recovery day.

-Thai Cucumber salad and Tom Kha Gai

1 English cucumber OR 2 field cucumbers (if using organic, leave the skin on; otherwise, wash well or peel it off)

1 shallot, minced (OR substitute 1/4 cup minced purple onion)

2 green (spring) onions, finely sliced

1 fresh red chili, de-seeded and minced fine, OR 1/4 cup diced red bell pepper

1/2 cup fresh coriander/cilantro, roughly chopped

1/4 cup ground or roughly chopped nuts of choice (not peanuts)

Dressing

2 Tbsp. fish sauce

juice of 1/2 lime

1-2 cloves garlic, minced

1/2 tsp. shrimp paste (available by the jar at Asian stores)

1 Tbsp. non-soy soy sauce alternative

1/4 to 1/2 tsp. cayenne pepper (to taste)

1 to 1+1/2 tsp. sugar

Cut the cucumber in half lengthwise, then repeat with each half until you have a number of long strips. Now slice the other way to create bite-size rectangular chunks. Place in a salad bowl.

Add the shallot, green onion, chili/red pepper, and coriander to the salad bowl (keep back a little extra coriander for a garnish).

Combine the dressing ingredients together in a cup, stirring to dissolve the shrimp paste. Taste-test it for sweet-sour balance, adding more sugar if it's too sour for your taste.

Pour dressing over the salad and toss well.

Top with the ground/chopped nuts, plus extra coriander. If desired, garnish with a slice of lime. Serve immediately, or cover and refrigerate for up to 3 hours.

Tom Kha Gai

1 quart chicken broth
1 can of coconut milk
1/4 tsp dried chile flakes
1 tsp freshly grated ginger
juice of 1 lemon
sea salt (to taste)
2 C cubed cooked chicken (optional)
2 green onions, chopped (optional)
chopped cilantro (optional)

Bring the stock to a boil, skim any foam that rises to the top and add coconut milk, lemon juice, chile flakes, ginger, and optional chicken. Simmer for about 15 minutes. Season to taste with salt. Ladle into soup bowls or mugs and garnish with cilantro and green onions.

1 serving is a medium-large bowl of soup and 1-2 cups of salad.

-Shrimp Sushi Salad

Marinated Shrimp

12 Shrimps pealed and deveined □ (may need to add more depending on # of people you're feeding)

5 tbsp sesame oil□

5 tbsp soy sauce□alternative

2 tbsp rice vinegar□

1 clove garlic□

1/2 red chili□2-inch

2 tsp fresh ginger, peeled and minced

Making the marinade: Mix the ingredients for the marinade in a bowl and add the shrimp. Make sure the marinade covers all of the Shrimp. Put in the fridge for 4-8 hours. Place the shrimp on a baking sheet and broil the shrimp. This should take no longer than 2-5 min. Shrimp turns pink when it is done. After you are done with the marinade cook it on a medium heat until it boils. Then let it cool and use it as the dressing.

White Rice, Brown Rice and/or Quinoa

Cook 1 cup of White Rice, Brown Rice and/or Quinoa

2 Tbs rice vinegar

1 tsp sesame oil

Combine ingredients

Salad

Marinated and cooked shrimp

White Rice, Brown Rice and/or Quinoa

1 large broccoli, broken into 1-inch pieces

- 1 green onion

- 2 avocado, cut into cubes

- 12 mushrooms (shiitake or

	whatever you prefer), cut in quarters
	☐ 1 handful sugarsnap peas, divided in half☐
	1 handful bean sprouts☐
	1/2 cucumber, cut into sticks☐
	8 sheets nori seaweed, cut into 2×2-inch squares
	☐ 1 handful roasted sesame seeds☐
	1 handful cilantro
	Blanch the broccoli (pour boiled water over it, let it set for two minutes and then throw it in ice cold water). Divide the rice into large bowls and top it with all the vegetables mixed together. Drizzle the rest of the marinade over the salad, top it with sesame seeds and cilantro and serve it with wasabi and soy sauce alternative. 1 serving is the equivalent of a medium to large bowl with 5-6 shrimp on it.
Post-workout Snack (only necessary after	-1-1.5 cups Kombucha with 1 avocado, salt and pepper to taste. We teach you how to make your own Kombucha, coconut milk, etc. inside http://www.bengreenfieldfitness.com/innercircle

workouts of 1+ hour in duration)	-1 large handful macadamia nuts or Brazil nuts if you haven't already had some earlier, with equivalent of 1 piece of fresh, raw fruit -1 scoop Supergreens in 1 cup whole coconut milk -1 Cocochia bar
Snack 3 (only necessary during workouts of 2+ hours in duration – you can also refer to "long workout fueling" section towards end of this book)	**Energy Gels –**150-300 calories//hr **Energy Drink –** 150-300 calories/hr of a sports electrolyte drink
Snack 4 (Post-workout within 60 minutes, only for	**¾-1 cup Yogurt + 1-2 handful dried fruits mixed with nuts** **Sweet potato** - 1 medium-large size with 1-2 tablespoons almond butter

workouts of 1+ hour in duration)	**1-2 Bars** – <u>Cocochia bar</u>

Fruit – 1 piece fresh and raw with 1-2 handfuls almonds or walnuts

Yam + chicken – 1 medium-large size with 4-6oz chicken breast

Quinoa– 1-2 cups (can season with salt/pepper or cinnamon/raisins) |
| **Supplements:** | -3 <u>Enerprime</u> in the morning, before breakfast. Work up to 6 over the course of 2 weeks. Alternative would be 2 tablespoons <u>Capragreens</u>.

-2 Fish Oil in the morning, with breakfast and 2 more in the evening, with dinner.

-3000-6000 IU per day of <u>Vitamin D3</u>, preferably using the nanospray.

-<u>Magnetic Clay Magnesium Oil</u>. 5 sprays applied topically to each forearm prior to workouts, and 5 sprays applied topically to each leg after workouts. <u>Natural Calm magnesium</u> (250-500mg) before bed.

-<u>Recoverease</u> (or other proteolytic enzymes source) 4-6 per day, preferably immediately after workout or later in day on an empty stomach. |

Again, if you must get quick nutrition and don't have time to cook, 2-3 heaping scoops of the Living Fuel SuperGreens mixed in ½ cup whole coconut milk or water can be used as a meal replacement for ANY of the meals on this plan. For an even lower carbohydrate option, such as when you are sitting at the office or late at night, the same substitution can be made, but with Living Fuel SuperProtein or DEEP30 protein.

Optional Supplements:

-5-10 Master Amino Pattern (or other whole amino acid) capsules prior to hard workouts

-Anytime you feel sick or get exposed to cold/flu, 5-6 drops of Oil of Oregano, taken under the tongue or in a glass of water, every night to eliminate any yeast or fungus.

Questions about supplements? Leave a support ticket at http://www.support.bengreenfieldfitnes s.com

-Probiotics/Digestive Enzymes. Check http://pacificfit.net/nutritional-

	<u>supplements</u> for Caprobiotics and Caprazymes.

Meal Plan For Biggest Training Day Of Week

This is the meal plan that you will eat for 1 day of the week, preferably your biggest, hardest day of training (for most, this falls on a weekend). While this isn't a full-on "cheat day", it certainly includes a higher caloric intake and less "clean eating" than the other days of the week.

You will not see any nutritional supplements on this meal plan, but you can continue to take the supplements you were taking the other 6 days of the week.

Breakfast (choose 1)	1. **Power Cereal** - ½-1 cup cooked quinoa or gluten-free oatmeal with 2-3 scoops protei⌐ , 2-4 tablespoons coconut ⌐ ⌐oon of ground fl⌐⌐ ⌐ablespoon ⌐iced banana. ⌐hoose 1 from list n. Add 2 scoops **⌐omato breakfast** ⌐es of gluten-free ⌐ wrap and eat avocado, a ⌐d a whole sliced 1 cup coconut

	milk
	4. Pancakes: To ¾-1 cup (preferably) gluten-free flour or almond flour, add ½ teaspoon baking powder, 2-4 tablespoons whole coconut milk, 1 egg, 1 scoop rice, pea or hemp protein powder (i.e. LivingProtein), 1 teaspoon vanilla, 1 teaspoon cinnamon and 1-2 tablespoons raw honey. Add water to desired texture. Grill with coconut oil or butter.
	5. Bread with berry spread – Spread two slices gluten free bread or a gluten free wrap with one handful of fresh raspberries, strawberries, or blueberries. Add 1 handful of pumpkin seeds, walnuts or almonds. Serve with 2 scoops protein stirred into 4-6 ounces coconut milk.
	6. Restaurant – hash browns or stack of pancakes + eggs and bacon.
Snack 1	**1 piece fruit** – recommend grapefruit, handful blueberries, pear or green apple. **1 cup shake** – see list at end of meal plan 1 **energy bar or snack mix** –

recommend the Cocochia bar or Cocochia Snack Mix. These are gluten-free, and a much more stable source of energy than most brands.

Bell pepper and jicama strips with hummus (store-bought or homemade is fine – 200-250 calories of hummus). How to make your own hummus: Blend 1 and ½ cups of garbanzo beans, ½ cup tahini, 3 tablespoons olive oil, 1-2 shallots, ½ teaspoon of sea salt, ½ teaspoon cumin, ½ teaspoon black pepper, ½ cup lemon juice, 2 tablespoon chopped parsley and a pinch of paprika. Serve a ½ cup sized portion with 1/2 sliced red and green pepper or 5-6 slices of jikama. Refrigerate the remainder. Add cayenne pepper for a metabolic boost. *To improve digestibility, prior to cooking, soak the garbanzo beans for up to 24 hours and add just a bit of vinegar in the soaking solution.*

1 handful snack mix

Lunch– choose 1 (can use kelp, kombu, or dulse	**Wrap:** For outer wrap, use gluten free wrap. You could also use kale, bok choy or some other large, dark leafy green, and then just include a brown or white rice inside wrap. For meat, use 4-6oz turkey, chicken, ground beef, ground

seasoning)	buffalo, or non-fried fish. For vegetable options, use avocado, peppers, cucumber, tomato, sprouts, red onion, or celery. For sauce or dressing options, use olive oil/vinaigrette, lemon or lime juice, or a soy sauce alternative or a mix of all three. **Turkey Avocado Sandwich or Wrap.** Use two slices gluten-free bread or wrap, 3-4 slices preservative-free, sodium-free deli turkey, 1/2-1 avocado, ½-1 tomato, 1 large handful dark leafy greens like spinach or kale. **Cashew Stir Fry:** Cook 1 cup rice, quinoa, amaranth or millet according to package directions. Sautee vegetables in 1 tbs. sesame oil or coconut oil, adding: 1/2 sliced bell pepper, 1 tsp. grated ginger root, 1 grated lime rind, 2 sliced shallots, 1 grated carrot, 1 handful sugar-snap peas, 1 handful sliced mushrooms, 1 handful broccoli, 1 handful cashews, & 1/2 sliced cucumber. Spice with a pinch of turmeric & curry, then salt/pepper to taste. Serve 1-2 handfuls vegetable mix over ½-1 cup cooked starch. **Leftovers**: 1 serving from dinner
Snack 2	**1 Handful Snack Mix** – Choose 1 from list

	Guacamole: Blend ½ avocado and stir in a chopped ½ red or green pepper, ½ chopped tomato, ½ teaspoon cumin, and a sprinkling of cayenne pepper. Serve with a 2-3 handfuls of gluten-free crackers, rice crackers or corn chips. 1 **energy bar** – recommend the <u>Cocochia bar</u> or <u>Cocochia Snack Mix</u>.
Snack 3 (during workout for longer workouts – or refer to "long workout fueling" section towards end of this book)	**Energy Gels** –200-300 calories/hr **Or** **Energy Drink –** 200-300 calories/hr of a sports electrolyte drink **Or (this is lowest carb option)** 30-60 minutes prior: 1g sodium (i.e. a chicken boullion cube – this keeps your blood pressure high enough on a low carb intake), 5-10g BCAA's or EAA's (I recommend 10 Master Amino Pattern capsules - <u>MAP</u>) and 2-3 tablespoons <u>medium chain triglyceride oil</u> or <u>coconut oil</u>. Every hour during workout: 5g <u>BCAA's</u> or <u>EAA's</u> (such as 5 <u>MAP</u> capsules per hour) and 100-150 calories <u>UCAN SuperStarch</u>

	per hour. Also - optional, but discussed more in the supplementary chapter at the end of this book - 1 serving <u>VESPA per hour.</u>
Snack 4 (Post-workout within 20-60 minutes)	**1 cup shake** – Choose 1 from list **1 Handful Snack Mix** – Choose 1 from list **Sweet potato** - 1 medium-large size with 1 tablespoon almond butter **1 Bar** – <u>Cocochia bar</u> **Fruit** – 1 piece fresh and raw with 1-2 handfuls almonds or walnuts **Yam + chicken** – 1 medium-large size with 4-6oz chicken breast **Quinoa** – 250-350 calories (can season with salt/pepper or cinnamon/raisins)
Dinner	**Beer Can Chicken and Black Quinoa & Kale salad** Beer Can Chicken 1 (4 lbs) Whole Chicken 2 Tbl coconut oil or grape seed oil 2 Tbl salt 1 tsp black pepper 3 Tbl of your favorite dry spice rub

1 can of beer

Remove neck and giblets from chicken and discard. Rinse chicken inside and out, and pat dry with paper towels. Rub chicken lightly with oil then rub inside and out with salt, pepper and dry rub. Set aside.

Open a beer can and poor out half or drink half whatever you prefer. Place beer can on a rimmed baking sheet. Place the chicken cavity over the beer can.

Cook the chicken on 350 for approximately 1 1/4 hours or until the internal temperature registers 165 degrees F in the breast area and 180 degrees F in the thigh, or until the thigh juice runs clear when stabbed with a sharp knife. Remove from oven and let rest for 10 minutes before carving.

Black Quinoa & Kale Salad

1 ½ cup black quinoa cooked and cooled

Dressing

4 Tbl olive oil
½ organic lemon (peal and juice)

2 Tbl hot mustard
salt and pepper to tast

Salad

4 big leafs of Kale
2 apples
1 handful of sprouts
1 cup of feta cheese

Cook the quinoa. Mix the ingredients for the dressing in a high glass or a small bowl. Let the quinoa cool off for a while and add the dressing. Rinse the kale and chop it. Cut the apples in small cubes. Mix all the ingredients with the quinoa and top it with the goat cheese. Eat until full.

Barley Bean Soup

3 tbsp olive oil

2 spring onions, chopped

3 cloves garlic, chopped

3 small carrots, diced

2 ribs celery, diced

2 tsp fresh rosemary, chopped

□2 bay leaves (can be replaced with sage)

□juice from 1/2 lemon□

1/2 glass white wine□

8 cups vegetable stock

□1 cup pearled barley□

1 zucchini, cut in quarters

□10 cherry tomatoes, divided in half

□2 cups fresh green beans□

1 cup fresh or frozen beans and preboiled for 20 min.

Heat olive oil in a heavy-bottomed pot and add onion and garlic. Saute for about 5 minutes. Add carrots, celery, rosemary, bay leaves, lemon juice and white wine and cook, stirring often, for 2 minutes. Add vegetable stock and let it cook for 30 minutes. Add barley, zucchini, and tomatoes and let it cook for another 25 min. Then add green beans and borlotti beans and let it simmer for 10 more min. Remove the bay leaves and add salt and pepper. The soup is done when the barley and the beans are done. Serve with olive oil, lemon juice and fresh herbs.

Zucchini and Chickpeas salad and Pancetta and Turkey Meatloaf

Pancetta and Turkey Meatloaf (an adapted recipe from Giada De Laurentiis)
Ingredients

> 1/2 cup ground oats
> 1/4 cup chopped flat-leaf parsley
> 2 large eggs, lightly beaten
> 2 tablespoons whole milk
> 1/2 cup grated Romano or Pramesan
> 1/4 cup chopped sun-dried tomatoes
> 3/4 teaspoon salt
> 3/4 teaspoon freshly ground black pepper
> 1 pound ground turkey, preferably dark meat
> 10 ounces sliced pancetta, about 10 slices or you can use bacon

Preheat the oven to 375 degrees F.

In a large bowl, stir together the bread crumbs, parsley, eggs, milk, cheese, sun-dried tomatoes, salt, and pepper. Add the turkey and gently stir to combine, being careful not to overwork the meat.

On a baking sheet lined with parchment paper, lay out the pancetta, overlapping the slices, into a large rectangle shape. In the middle of the rectangle, place the turkey mixture, shaping into a loaf. Using the parchment paper, wrap the pancetta up and around the turkey loaf to cover completely. Squeeze the parchment-covered loaf with your hands to secure the pancetta and solidify the shape of the loaf. While still covered in parchment, bake the loaf until the internal temperature reaches 165 degrees F on an instant-read thermometer, about 45 minutes. Remove from the oven and let cool.

Zucchini and Chickpeas salad

Dressing

> 2 Tbl fresh lemon juice
> ¼ cup Olive oil
> ½ tsp salt
> ¼ tsp pepper

combine all ingredients

Salad
> 1 cup cooked garbanzo bean

2 medium zucchini, cut into ¼ in pieces

½ cup frozen corn thawed

½ small red onion thinly sliced

1 red bell pepper diced

1 oz parmesan cubed into ¼ in pieces

Place the garbanzo beans, zucchini, corn, red onion, and lettuce in a large salad bowl. Pour the vinaigrette over the salad and toss well garnish with the crumbled Parmesan cheese and serve. Eat until full.

Black Bean Flautas and Mexican Cabbage salad

Black Bean Flautas

2 tsp. coconut oil

1 medium onion, chopped (about 1 cup)

2 cloves garlic, minced (about 2 tsp.)

2 cups black beans

2 tsp. chili powder

1 16-oz. tub prepared salsa, divided

1 cup fresh or frozen corn kernels

12 6-inch sprouted wheat tortillas

1/4 cup chopped cilantro

Heat oil in skillet over medium heat. Cook onion 3 to 5 minutes, or until soft. Add garlic, and cook 1 minute, or until translucent and fragrant.

Stir in beans, chili powder and 1 cup water. Reduce heat to medium low, and simmer 10 minutes, or until most of liquid has evaporated. Remove from heat. Mash beans until mixture is thickened but still chunky, and some beans remain whole. Stir in 1 cup salsa and corn, and season with salt and pepper. Cool.

Preheat oven to 425F. Coat 2 large baking sheets with cooking spray. Spoon 1/3 cup black bean mixture down center of tortilla. Roll tortilla around filling, and secure closed with toothpick. Set on prepared baking sheet. Repeat with remaining tortillas and black bean mixture. Bake 6 to 10 minutes, or until tortillas are browned and crisp.

Meanwhile, combine cilantro and remaining salsa in small bowl. Place 2 flautas on each plate, and top with remaining salsa.

Mexican Cabbage Salad

Salad

1/2 head large cabbage, shredded
1/2 cup fresh cilantro, chopped
1/4 cup fresh mint, chopped
1 medium cucumber, chopped

Honey Lime Dressing

Juice of 1 lime
1/4 cup olive oil
2 Tbl raw honey
2 tbsp finely chopped cilantro
1 garlic clove, peeled and minced (or 1 medium shallot, minced)
1/2 tsp kosher salt
Freshly ground pepper

Combine ingredients and shake very well. Toss Salad. Eat until full.

Restaurant: Splurge at your favorite restaurant. Order a non-fried meat, vegetables and starch of your choice. Try to avoid things that were cooked in vegetables oils, or a high amount on non-nutrient dense starches (i.e. going to a Mexican restaurant and mowing

	through two baskets of fried chips). Fine to eat until full on this day.
Desserts and Cheat Meals (consume before, during or after exercise only, preferably only 3 days of the week)	1 Handful Frozen Fruit with ½ cup Yogurt with 1TBS raw honey 1 150-200 calorie Dark Chocolate Bar dipped in 1TBS Almond Butter Almond Butter/Chocolate Protein Shake (1TBS Almond or Cashew Butter + 1 scoop protein powder, + 1 TBS hershey's chocolate, ½ banana (optional), and ice/water to taste) 1 Handful Almonds or Walnuts drizzled with Honey – sautee nuts in 1 teaspoon olive oil for 5-10 minutes, lightly add sea salt, and drizzle with 1TBS raw honey. Reese's Cup: Use ½-1 cup of plain yogurt, or coconut milk. Add 1 tablespoon nut butter and 1 tablespoon dark chocolate pieces or cocoa mix. Stir together, close your eyes and imagine you just took it out of that little orange wrapper. Freeze for added effect.

Snack mix recipes:

Berry Almond Snack Mix: Mix at beginning of week: 2 cups almonds, 1 cup dried cherries or blueberries, 1 cup flax seeds. Keep in freezer.

Sunny Seed Mix (highest in Iron): Mix at beginning of week: 3 cups sunflower seeds, 1 cup sesame seeds, 1 cup pumpkin seeds, 1 cup flax seeds. Keep in freezer.

Tropical Snack Mix (also very high in Iron): Mix at beginning of week: 2 cups raw coconut shavings (preferably unsweetened), 2 cups raisins or craisins, 2 cups Brazil nuts, 1 cup dried mango or chopped papaya and 1 cup flax seeds. Keep in freezer.

Shake recipes: For higher calories or post-workout shakes, highly recommend adding 10-20 grams of LivingProtein or DEEP30.

Blueberry coconut shake - Combine a handful of frozen blueberries, 3 tablespoons of shredded, unsweetened coconut and ice to desired texture. Add approx 4oz unsweetened coconut milk, almond milk, rice milk or water to desired texture and blend.

Nutty shake– Combine 1 tablespoon almond butter, 2 tablespoons shredded, unsweetened coconut, 2 tablespoons sunflower seeds, ice and water or 4oz unsweetened coconut milk, almond milk or rice milk.

Coconut-Kiwi: Blend together 4oz unsweetened coconut milk, almond milk, rice milk or water, ½ cup frozen apricots or peaches, and 1 frozen kiwi.

Berry shake - Combine a handful of frozen berries and ice to desired texture. Add 4oz unsweetened coconut milk, almond milk, rice milk or water and blend.

Nutty banana shake – Combine 2 tablespoons flax seeds, 1 handful almonds or walnuts, 1 banana and ice to desired texture. Add 4oz unsweetened coconut milk, almond milk, rice milk or water.

Long Workout "Real Food" Options

Important: when I say "Long Workout", I'm referring to workouts that are A) aerobic; B) 2+ hours and 3) not an effort for which speed is a primary goal. An example would be a multi-day bike ride, a day hike, a long, slow trail run, etc.

These are the type of workouts you'd do during base training for an Ironman, during some type of endurance camp, or for a long social workout.

The goal is to consume 150-300 calories per hour if you are female or a small individual or 250-400 calories per hour if you are male or a large individual, and to get these from sources that are not pure sugar. Choices are:

-2-3 handfuls of snack mix per hour (see earlier in this plan)

-Chia seed/water mix– 24-32 ounces per hour.

> *Put 1/3 cup of dry chia seeds into a 32 ounce Nalgene bottle, or other water bottle.*

> *Fill the Nalgene with water 1/3 of the way and then pour chia seeds into the water.*

Close the lid tightly and shake the bottle, then open the bottle and fill it with water the rest of the way. Close the lid and shake again.

To prevent lumps from forming, shake about every 5 minutes.

Add Stevia and Lemon if desired for sweetness.

-Carob Cashew bars – 2-3/hr

1 c. cashew butter
3 tbsp. honey
1 1/2 c. protein powder (Mt. Capra Double Bonded works well for this)
1 c. old fashioned oats
1 tbsp. carob powder
Mix the cashew butter and honey in a bowl, and heat for 30 seconds (use a saucepan, or in a pinch, a microwave). Add the rest of ingredients and mix together. Mixture should be crumbly. Press (hard) into a 9x9 tray and refrigerate for 20 minutes. Cut into bars.

-Chocolate Almond Butter "Rollies" – equivalent of 1-2 wraps per hour

Spread 1 tablespoon of almond butter, 1 teaspoon honey and 2 tablespoons carob chips or chocolate chips into a sprouted wrap, roll up, and chop into bite size pieces. Carry in aluminum foil.

When it comes to eating real food during a workout, there are multitude of other options, but these are some of my favorites, and hopefully they get your wheels turning!

Race Week

Up to the point where you reach the week of your big event, you have been on a fairly low carbohydrate intake, but you don't want to go into your event in a state of storage carbohydrate (glycogen) depletion.

For that reason, about 5-6 days prior to your event you need to gradually begin refueling with more carbohydrate. Let's use a Sunday race as an example.

Beginning Monday or Tuesday, add the equivalent of one large sweet potato or yam with breakfast. I'd recommend you do this with an egg based meal, and of course, adding in a liberal amount of vegetables until 2 days before the race, at which point you will need to begin limiting fiber intake.

Also beginning Monday or Tuesday, with a salad at lunch, include a side of 3/4-1 cup cooked brown rice, white rice, or mashed sweet potato/yam. Salt and pepper to taste, and if you'd like, you can even boil or roast vegetables and serve those over the rice instead of having a cold salad.

Since you are likely going to be done with your workouts at night and ready to be primarily sedentary, dinner should continue to be primarily protein and vegetable based until the night before the race. Rather than putting the extra carbohydrate with dinner, you should put it with breakfast and lunch and then *after your race week workouts.*

After your primary workout of the day each day during race week, consume one large piece of fresh raw fruit of your choice OR the equivalent of 1 cooked sweet potato or yam (I recommend you do either of these with 6-8 <u>Recoverease</u>) OR 2 handfuls of berries of your choice blended with ice and 1-2 scoops protein powder.

The night before your race, choose a dark meat of your choice (4-6 oz steak or salmon), since dark meat will have higher iron and mitochondria content. Combine this with a small side of dark leafy greens, such as steamed and salted spinach, along with a hearty serving of quinoa, brown rice, white rice, baked potato, sweet potato, or yam. You should be consuming about 400-600 calories of carbohydrate with this meal.

The next morning, your pre-race meal, as you have probably guessed, should be a complex carbohydrate that is easily digested – and my top recommendation is 1-2 medium-large sweet potatoes or yams with salt, 1 tablespoon honey or maple syrup, and a dab of almond butter. Try to have this meal completely finished at least 2 hours and no more than 3 hours before the race begins.

Sound simple?

It actually is. All you're doing is replacing a few of your primarily fat and protein based meals with carbohydrates.

Finally, you do not need to do the "hard workout", "carbohydrate loading" day on race week. Your other modifications will take care of your carbohydrate stores.

If you are a caffeine user, then please try to switch to decaf or Teeccino 7-10 days prior to the race.

Race day (from 2011 version)

The version of race day fueling you are about to read is from the original 2011 release of this book. Below it is a more updated version using what I feel to be an even better scenario. But I didn't want to remove the original version because it still works very well for many people!

Because I practice what I preach, I'm going to give you an example of exactly what I do on race day during my Half-Ironman and Ironman events. Why those distances? Because, frankly, you don't need to eat anything at all during a Sprint triathlon, and I can sum up Olympic distance fueling in one sentence:

> *Eat a gel right before the swim starts, then consume 200-300 calories per hour of an electrolyte sports drink like Hammer HEED or GU Brew on the bike, mixed into 24-28oz of water per hour, and finish with a gel every 30 minutes on the run.*

Easy enough?

OK, let's move on to the long days, where fueling is much more crucial and your body's carbohydrate stores are much more likely to be fully depleted.

Remember that on race day, your goal is not to lose weight or engage in the low carbohydrate eating patterns you've been doing on a weekly basis, but rather to give your body high-octane, race day fuel.

Instead, assuming your race is a high-priority event, you will want to allow yourself to maintain as high an intensity as possible, and this means you'll need primarily carbohydrate based fuels. But if you've done everything right up to this point, your body will be highly equipped to use fat as efficiently as possible, ensuring that you tap into your body's storage carbohydrate much less quickly.

Ready for the rundown? OK, here we go.

- Between the time you eat breakfast 2-3 hours prior to the race and the actual start of the race, consume 20-24 ounces of water per hour, and taper that water intake off about 30 minutes before the race starts.

- 30-60 minutes prior to the race, consume any supplements that you take for sports performance. For me, this would include deltaE, Energy28, NutraRev, and MAP.

- 5-10 minutes prior to the race, consume a gel, preferably the type with caffeine. I personally use GU Roctane, which has amino acids in it that prevent fatigue and post-workout soreness.

- When you come out of the swim, consume 15-20 ounces plain water, along with 2-4 electrolytes (I recommend Athlytes by Millennium Sports) and 100-200 additional calories (e.g. 1-2 more gels).

- On the bike, consume 24-32 ounces of water per hour (volume depends on race conditions), 2-4 electrolyte capsules per hour, and 250-450 calories of amino acid containing gel or solids per hour (choose higher quantity for larger males). I personally do 3 GU Roctanes per hour (2 of those non-caffeinated), along with half a bag of GU Chomps at the end of each hour. This will definitely mean that you'll have extra fuel in your bike special needs bag if you don't want to be carrying all those gels.

- On the run, you can continue to use your own gels, such as the GU Roctane, or switch to the gels at the aid stations on the course if you do not prefer to carry your own nutrition. In both distances, you will not be able to eat as much on the run. For both the half-marathon and marathon in these races, you should consume 200-300 calories per hour (a gel ever 20-30 minutes), along with continued use of 2-4 electrolyte capsules per hour. Water volume should also decrease to 15-20 ounces of water per hour.

Does this also sound simple?

That's because it is.

Too many folks make things way too complex for Ironman race day nutrition. If you keep things simple, you'll know exactly how much you've had to eat and drink, and when you've had it, and this will help you tremendously with adhering to your race day nutrition plan.

I would give you precise post-race nutrition and recovery recommendations, but this would be mildly hypocritical, since I am usually the guy with a steak and a martini post-race. However, if you want my more serious thoughts on a speedy post-Ironman recovery, then click here to read my free article on lightning speed post-Ironman recovery secrets.

Race Day (Updated Version)

In 2012, I developed the following healthy, low carb race day nutrition protocol, designed to utilize fatty acids, stabilize blood sugars, and reduce post-race gas and bloating. This is the exact protocol I practiced with and used successfully to win long races.

1) High Molecular Weight Carbohydrate.

Glucose, sucrose, fructose, and maltodextrin are all sugars that cause a sudden flood of insulin to the body by way of the pancreas. While this is less of an issue when you're in an insulin sensitive state (such as when you're exercising or racing), when you consume these forms of sugar you still experience a constant spiking and dropping of blood sugar, *in addition to to the fermentation issues that you just learned about.*
As a result, you get frequent spikes and drops in energy during a race, and also post-race bloating and stomach issues.

So the first tier of my healthy race day nutrition plan was to find a slow-time release source of energy that allowed me to eat less, tap into my body's own fatty acid stores more efficiently, and not cause post-race gut rot.

Enter UCAN SuperStarch, which was originally developed as a slowly metabolized starch that would allow people with a rare condition called "Glycogen Storage Disease" to be able to have access to a very stable source of glucose.

UCAN is a high molecular weight, corn-derived starch that is metabolized differently than simpler sugars such as fructose or maltodextrin. It is a powder that you mix with water, and it's metabolism results in far less insulin production and less blood sugar spiking compared to other gels and sports drinks, and as a result of these lower insulin levels, this approach also allows your body to tap into it's own storage fat as a fuel.

How I used UCAN: I simply consumed 2 servings (220 calories) 2 hours before the race, then 2 servings per hour during the entire 3 hour bike and 1 hour run. I mixed 6 packets (enough for 3 hours) into a water bottle that I kept on the downtube of my bicycle and consumed a mouthful every half hour, and put 2 packets in a flask that I "nursed" on the run.

2) Flavor & Energy Boost

One drawback to UCAN is that most of it is flavored with artificial sweeteners, so I choose the plain, unsweetened version. But the plain version tastes a bit "chalky". So I wanted to figure out a way to add a bit of flavor, and also get some extra energy-boosting compounds.

Enter Energy28 Liquid Superfood. It's primary components are:

-Rhodiola rosea – a popular plant in traditional medical systems in Russia and Scandinavian countries for centuries, with a reputation for stimulating the nervous system, enhancing work performance and eliminating fatigue. *This came in quite handy, as this race occurred at 5000 feet elevation.*

-Organic Peruvian maca - a root vegetable, shaped like a radish, that grows high in the harsh climate of the Andes Mountains in South America at elevations up to 15,000 feet. Native Peruvians have used maca as a high-energy food and cortisol stabilizer for more than two millennia. Maca is high in vitamins as well as calcium, magnesium, potassium and other minerals.

-D-ribose – used by all the body's cells and essential in energy metabolism. Our bodies make ribose innately, but our cells lack the ability to produce it fast enough or in sufficient quantity to effectively offset the loss of energy from our cells.

-Golden Chlorella – a unique nutrient-dense, ultra-pure, mild-tasting microalgae that provides naturally occurring amino acids, vitamins and minerals. It is a complete functional food containing 50 percent omega 3, 6 and 9 oils by weight.

While there are some trace amounts of fructose from these superfood extracts in Energy28, there is still far, far less than what I was getting from the typical gel, chews, bars, or sports drink combo, and I found that the flavor of Energy28 gave the UCAN SuperStarch a pleasant, slightly fruity taste.

How I used Energy28: I simply consumed 1 serving for each serving of UCAN. So I put 6 servings in the water bottle that I had the UCAN in, and 2 servings in the flask of UCAN that I carried on the run.

3) Amino Acids

As I've written about extensively in this 2 part series on amino acids, high blood levels of amino acids primarily:

1) reduce your rating of perceived exertion, allowing you to work harder without your brain "shutting down" your body;

2) keep your body from cannibalizing your own lean muscle during exercise, thus limiting post-workout or post-race soreness.

But most proteins (the source of amino acids) need to be digested, which can take a long time and shuttle a lot of extra blood away from your muscles and into your stomach. Enter Master Amino Pattern (MAP).

MAP is a unique blend of 8 essential amino acids that collectively have a Body Protein Synthesis (BPS) of Net Nitrogen Utilization (NNU) that is 99% per 23 minutes.

Compared to MAP, something like a whey or soy protein source has a BPS/min of 16-32% NNU/180-360 min. This means that the BPS/min of a protein supplement is 24 to 96 times lower compared to MAP.

In a nutshell, the MAP capsules completely digest in 23 minutes, while other protein sources take anywhere from 2-6 hours. While a low, slow release source of protein might be OK for breakfast or before you go to bed at night, during exercise you want readily available sources of amino acids that don't need to undergo breakdown and digestion.

How I used Master Amino Pattern (MAP): I consumed 10 capsules 30 minutes prior to the race, then simply carried a small ziplock bag of MAP in my shorts and ate 5 per hour during the entire bike ride.

And that's it. That was my healthy race day nutrition protocol.

The result?
Despite eating far less than normal during the race, my energy levels were elevated the entire time – without having to force down sickeningly sweet gels. No crashes, no bonks, no burp-ups.

And better yet: *I had zero embarrassing post-race gas issues.*

Rather than you having to go the four corners of the planet to get this stuff, I figured out how to just bundle it all for you in 1 convenient Low Carb Fueling package:
http://goo.gl/Yryi5 <–UCAN+MAP+Energy28 Low Carb Fueling Package

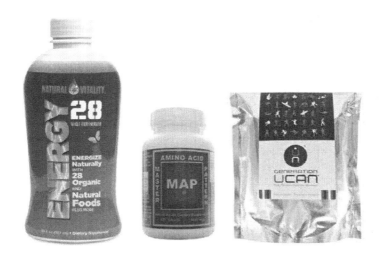

The package above is basically 60 packets of UCAN, a full 120 tablet bottle of MAP & a bottle of Energy28 – everything you need to get your low carb fueling dialed in, and about 1-2 months worth of fueling!

Possible additions to the scenario above:

If you're new to low carb fueling and struggle with dizziness from low blood pressure or lack of energy, 30-60 minutes prior to the race or training session in which you practice this fueling scenario: 1g sodium (i.e. a chicken boullion cube – this keeps your blood pressure high enough on a low carb intake), 5-10g BCAA's or EAA's (I recommend 10 Master Amino

Pattern capsules - <u>MAP</u>) and 2-3 tablespoons <u>medium chain triglyceride oil</u> or <u>coconut oil</u>.

Also - optional, but discussed more in the supplementary chapter at the end of this book - 1 serving <u>VESPA per hour.</u>

7 Supplements That Help You Perform Better On A Low Carbohydrate Diet

Since the original publishing of this book, I've written several articles on my blog about how to practically implement a low carbohydrate diet.

For example, I released the podcast: Is It Possible To Be Extremely Active and Eat A Low Carbohydrate Diet?

I've also produced these articles about how to avoid typical recommended carbohydrates dosages and instead eat a higher fat diet:

-Can You Build Muscle On A Low Carbohydrate Diet?

-Should You Eat Carbohydrates Before Exercise?

-How I Ate A High Fat Diet, Pooped 8 Pounds, And Then Won A Sprint Triathlon.

-The Hidden Dangers Of A Low Carbohydrate Diet

-10 Ways To Do A Low Carbohydrate Diet The Right Way

And Tim Olsen, the <u>winner of the brutal Western States 100 Mile Run, has just revealed that he is a low carb athlete</u>.

But the reality is that it can be very, very difficult and uncomfortable to switch to a low carbohydrate or "ketogenic" diet if you don't have the help of a few supplements – especially if you're serious about performance in sports like triathlon, Crossfit, marathoning and other high-energy depleting events.
So now I'm going to tell you about 7 supplements that can help you perform better on a low carbohydrate diet, along with a couple footnotes at the end that I think you'll find very interesting.

---

1. **Sodium**.

When you shift to a low carbohydrate or a ketogenic diet, your body loses storage carbohydrate, and also begins excreting sodium and water. When this happens, your blood pressure quickly drops, and much of the low energy that is attributed to "low blood sugar" when eating low carbohydrates is actually due to this low blood pressure.

Because of this, if you experience feelings of lightheadedness or sluggishness (especially during your workouts) you should include extra sodium in your diet. One strategy is to get 1-2g of extra sodium during the day by using vegetable or chicken bouillon cubes. I personally do fine by simply using 2-3 effervescent electrolyte tablets each day (I use the brand "nuun All-Day") combined with liberal use of sea salt on my meals.

You'll need to especially be sure to include extra sodium (close to 1g is good) about 30 minutes prior to your workout.

But if you already get 3-4g of sodium per day in your diet, this is probably a moot point for you.

Caveat: the extra sodium is not because Tim Noakes was wrong in my interview with him. You don't need extra electrolytes during your workout to keep your muscles from cramping. This is simply extra sodium to help you maintain adequate blood plasma volume and blood pressure.

---

2. Branched Chain Amino Acids.

In my podcast episode "Do Amino Acids Really Help You Exercise Or Are Nutrition Supplement Companies Just Pulling A Fast One On You", you learned about Branched Chain Amino Acids (BCAA's).

The BCAAs are unique from other amino acids because the enzymes responsible for their degradation are low in your tissues, so they appear rapidly in the blood stream, and expose your muscle to high concentrations – ultimately staving off muscle breakdown and stimulating muscle synthesis – even during exercise.

BCAA supplementation after exercise has been shown to cause faster recovery of muscle strength, and even more interestingly, the ability to slow down muscle breakdown – even during intense training and "overreaching" (getting very close to overtraining).

When you supplement with BCAA's, they can decrease the blood indicators of muscle tissue damage after long periods of exercise, thus indicating reduced muscle damage, and they also help maintain higher blood levels of amino acids, which can make you feel happy even when you're suffering during exercise.

But most importantly, if you're on a low carbohydrate diet, when taken prior to a fasted exercise session, BCAA's could improve your fat oxidation and utilization of storage fatty acids as a fuel.

Dosage for BCAA's would be leucine, isoleucine and valine in a 3g:1.5g:1.5g ratio. I personally just use whole amino acids (see below), but they're spendier, so if you want to go with BCAA's you could use the supplement Recoverease, at about 4 capsules an hour.

_____

3. **Whole Amino Acids**.

Whole amino acids offer you all the benefits of Branched Chain Amino Acids, and then some. Whole amino acids (also known as essential amino acids, or EAA's),were essentially (pun intended) summed up in this article I wrote previously about EAA's:

"If all 8 essential amino acids are present, muscle repair and recovery can start before you're even done with your workout – and when you're mentally stretched toward the end of a tough workout, game or race, high blood levels of amino acids can allow the body and brain to continue to work hard instead of shutting down."

This is all the more true if you're in a carbohydrate depleted state.

Anyways, protein quality is typically determined based on the EAA profile of any given protein, and generally, animal and dairy products contain the highest percentage of EAAs, resulting in greater protein synthesis and post-workout recovery than vegetarian protein-matched control.

But you don't have to take a steak (or your pea and rice protein powder blend) out with you on your workouts. Most of the clients I coach are now simply popping 5 Master Amino Pattern capsules during their long workouts or races, and getting extremely fast absorbing EAA's in the process.

<u>Master Amino Pattern</u> capsules are spendy, but if you want the best of AA's, this would be the way to go. 10 before very long workouts, then 5 every hour.

---

4. <u>Glutamine</u>.

Glutamine plays a role in muscle glycogen synthesis and whole-body carbohydrate storage. This was first observed in a study in the American Journal of Physiology that found that an infusion of glutamine promoted a resynthesis of muscle glycogen stores that wasn't observed in a control group infused with alanine plus glycine.

An oral dose of glutamine at about 8 grams can promote storage of muscle glycogen to levels similar to consuming straight glucose, which is especially useful when you don't have much glycogen (storage carbohydrate) to go around due to a low carbohydrate diet.

Glutamine supplementation has also been shown to enhance glucose production during exercise. Once again, if you're carbohydrate restricted in your diet, this can be good news. There's also some evidence that supplementation with glutamine may be effective for preventing immune suppression from strenuous exercise.

To use glutamine properly, you'd just take 8g of regular old glutamine immediately after your workout (avoid the glutamine powders with artificial sweeteners and additives).

---

5. Taurine.

In a study entitled "Potentiation of the actions of insulin by taurine", the amino acid taurine was shown to have a carbohydrate sparing effect. Taurine may also amplify the effect of insulin, allowing for more efficient carbohydrate utilization.

Research on taurine and caffeine containing beverages have shown that during prolonged endurance exercise, decreased heart rate and decreased catecholamine (stress hormones) are observed compared to using caffeine alone. Based on this, many folks will slam a Red Bull energy drink during a tough, long event.

But I don't recommend Red Bull, for a variety of reasons, including the presence of artificial sweeteners and citric acid. Instead, you can just do **2g of a taurine supplement, about 30-60 minutes prior to a tough or long exercise session in a relatively carbohydrate depleted state**.

---

6. Medium Chain Triglyceride Oil or Coconut Oil.

When you exercise while on a low carbohydrate diet, you're going to be burning lots of fatty acids as a fuel, and the medium chain triglycerides (MCT's) that you'll find in <u>medium chain triglyceride oil</u> and <u>coconut oil</u> can be a tremendous asset for keeping your energy levels high.

The stuff is easy to use: **just take 2-3 tablespoons of <u>coconut oil</u> or 2-3 doses of <u>medium chain triglyceride oil</u> about 30-60 minutes before you head out for a workout session.**
You could technically repeat this dosage every 2-3 hours during something like a long bike ride, but it can be logistically difficult and messy to carry oils (feel free to e-mail me at <u>ben@bengreenfieldfitness.com</u> if you have a good solution for this).

———————————————

7. **<u>Magnesium</u>**.

Although a low carbohydrate diet doesn't massively deplete magnesium in the same way that it does sodium, upon switching to a low-carb diet (especially when combined with intense exercise) many people experience nighttime leg cramping and more muscle discomfort during exercise, and this is likely due to low magnesium.

About <u>70% of people don't get anywhere near enough magnesium</u>, and if you're leaching magnesium with a combination of your sweating and a low carbohydrate diet, you're almost guaranteed to have some muscle twitching issues. Considering that over 300 enzymes require magnesium as a co-factor to make them work properly, it's a smart move to add magnesium into a low carbohydrate diet.

You can do about 300-500 milligrams of something like Natural Calm Magnesium before you go to bed at night (I find that this really helps me sleep better), and then 10-15 sprays of a topical magnesium on each leg immediately before your workout. Back off the total amount of magnesium you consume if you get loose stool.

_____

What's This About "VESPA"?

In the book "_Art & Science of Low Carbohydrate Performance_", Jeff Volek and Steve Phinney mention a supplement called VESPA.

VESPA is basically a naturally-occuring amino acid compound that is extracted from wasps. The theory behind this supplement is that wasps rely upon this amino acid to be able to travel extremely far distances on relatively low amounts of carbohydrate fuel, and a relatively large reliance upon storage body fat.

While there's not much evidence on VESPA, there's plenty of anecdotes that it can give some benefit to people who are training in a low carbohydrate or ketogenic state.

For example, ultrarunner Tim Olsen just won the brutal Western States 100 Mile Running Race and said:

"_On race day, I use Vespa which is an amino acid supplement about every 2hrs and a 100 calorie gel pack about every hour. Being on a low carb diet helps me to efficiently burn fat as my fuel. The few cal an hour I use allow me to run as fast as I can..._"

I personally have not noticed a difference with VESPA when I used it with no other fuel sources, but in coming months, I will be experimenting with a combination of <u>VESPA</u>, <u>UCAN SuperStarch</u> and <u>Master Amino Pattern</u> during my long and hard training sessions. If I can sustain high speed and power output for long periods of time (e.g. a 3 hour Hammer-fest on the bike that I would normally need higher amounts of sugar to fuel) without gastrointestinal distress, I may end up using this approach in racing.

Summary

So you're gearing up for a killer exercise session, or a big event like a marathon or a triathlon...and you're eating a low carbohydrate diet, and not wanting to carbohydrate load or use lots of carbohydrate during the event.

Based on what I've written here, here's what you do:

30-60 minutes prior: 1g sodium (i.e. a chicken boullion cube), 5-10g BCAA's or EAA's, 2-3 tablespoons <u>medium chain triglyceride oil</u> or <u>coconut oil</u>, 2g <u>taurine</u> and 10-15 sprays <u>topical magnesium</u> on each limb.

Every hour: 5g <u>BCAA's</u> or <u>EAA's</u>, and then optional, but recommended if you're redlining for multiple hours, 90-120 calories <u>UCAN SuperStarch</u> + 1 serving <u>VESPA</u>

Immediately after: 8g <u>glutamine</u>

Closing Thoughts

If you've made it this far in the guide, then you know more than 99% of the endurance athlete population when it comes to fueling your body for the combination of ideal health and performance, and you're ready for weight loss, longevity and breaking the sugar addiction.

So now is the time for you to head out to the trenches and start implementing what you've learned. Visit the grocery store. Reboot your pantry and refrigerator. Make it through those first 2 "uncomfortable" weeks. Go!

If you have questions about what you've read in this guide, then you have a few options.

For a one-time Q&A, just throw a question over to the free podcast at http://www.bengreenfieldfitness.com. You can ask a question using the "Ask Ben" form on any of the podcast shownotes, you can download the free iPhone or Android app and ask your question that way, or you can call 1-877-209-9439 and leave an audio question.

I also do personal consulting and one-on-one phone calls for more intensive Q&A or for more detailed conversations. To see your nutrition and exercise consulting options, just visit http://www.pacificfit.net

Ben Greenfield

About The Author

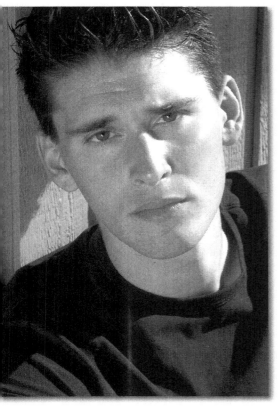

Ben Greenfield is a nationally recognized authority in sports nutrition, endurance sports training, fat loss, wellness and human performance.

Ben offers a free blog and podcast, which you can access by **clicking here**, and also offers personal, one-on-one nutrition and exercise consulting services to anyone, anywhere in the world, via **Pacific Elite Fitness.**

You can find all Ben's books by **clicking here.**

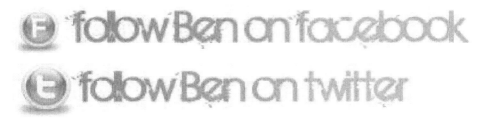

Made in the USA
Lexington, KY
05 March 2013